QUICK ACTION CHAIR YOGA FOR SENIORS.

A Routine Fitness Handbook for Seniors Health, Physical and Mental Wellbeing.

Table of Contents

CHAPTER ONE

INTRODUCTION

Chair yoga is a modified version of traditional yoga, specifically designed for individuals who can practice while sitting on a chair or using it for support. This form of yoga aims to extend the advantages of yoga to those with limited mobility, physical constraints, or difficulties in practicing on the floor.

1.1 Key features of chair yoga include:

Accessibility: Chair yoga eliminates the need for floor-based poses, making it suitable for a diverse range of individuals, including seniors, those with disabilities, and individuals in recovery.

Gentle Movements: Chair yoga involves adapted stretches, twists, and movements that are gentle and suitable for a seated position. The focus is on enhancing flexibility, strength, and balance without causing stress to the joints.

Breath Awareness: Similar to traditional yoga, chair yoga incorporates mindfulness of breath. Practitioners are guided to synchronize their breathing with movements, fostering relaxation and mindfulness.

Improved Flexibility and Strength: Despite being seated, chair yoga targets various muscle groups, promoting flexibility and strength. This can contribute to increased mobility and overall physical well-being.

Mind-Body Connection: Chair yoga integrates mindfulness and meditation techniques, establishing a connection between the mind and body. This comprehensive approach can positively impact mental well-being, reducing stress and promoting a sense of calm.

Adaptability: Chair yoga can be practiced in various settings, such as the workplace, community centers, or at home. It requires minimal equipment, typically just a stable chair, making it a convenient and adaptable practice.

Chair yoga offers an accessible and inclusive way for people of all ages and physical abilities to enjoy the benefits of yoga. It provides a gentle and adaptable approach to enhancing physical health, mental well-being, and a feeling of equilibrium and relaxation.

1.2 Importance of Chair Yoga

Chair yoga is of great significance for seniors, providing a range of physical, mental, and emotional benefits tailored to the specific needs and challenges faced by older individuals. The practice is highly accessible, allowing seniors with limited mobility or physical constraints to engage in a form of exercise that is gentle and safe, eliminating the need for challenging floor-based poses. It incorporates gentle stretches and movements to enhance flexibility and joint mobility, addresses balance and stability, and emphasizes mindful breathing and relaxation techniques for stress reduction and improved mental well-being.

Moreover, chair yoga contributes to joint health by including exercises designed to alleviate stiffness and discomfort associated with conditions like arthritis. It also enables seniors to engage in strength-building exercises while seated, essential for maintaining muscle mass and functional strength. The practice fosters social interaction and a sense of community, offering seniors the opportunity to participate in a group activity. Additionally, chair yoga can be easily adapted to accommodate various health conditions commonly seen in seniors, such as cardiovascular issues, respiratory concerns, or osteoporosis, making it a versatile and inclusive practice.

Furthermore, chair yoga incorporates mindfulness and meditation, promoting a stronger mind-body connection, contributing to a positive outlook, improved focus, and a sense of inner calm. Overall, chair yoga plays a vital role in supporting seniors in maintaining or regaining independence in their daily lives, providing a safe, accessible, and enjoyable way for them to stay physically and mentally active as they age.

Chair yoga has transcended cultural boundaries and gained popularity on a global scale due to several factors that make it inclusive, adaptable, and accessible to people from diverse backgrounds:

Target Audience: Chair yoga is specifically designed for seniors, catering to individuals in the aging population who may have varying levels of mobility, flexibility, and physical abilities. This inclusive practice is suitable for those seeking a gentle and accessible form of exercise that can be done while seated.

Benefits of Chair Yoga for Seniors:

1. Improved Flexibility: Chair yoga helps seniors enhance their flexibility through gentle stretches and movements, promoting better joint mobility.

2. Enhanced Strength: Modified poses and resistance exercises in chair yoga contribute to improved muscle strength, supporting daily activities and reducing the risk of frailty.

3. Balance and Stability: The practice includes balancing poses that enhance stability, coordination, and reduce the risk of falls, promoting overall safety.

4. Stress Reduction: Mindful breathing and relaxation techniques incorporated in chair yoga contribute to stress reduction, fostering a sense of calm and mental well-being.

5. Joint Health: Chair yoga promotes joint health by incorporating movements that increase range of motion, reducing stiffness and discomfort often associated with aging.

6. Improved Posture: Emphasis on proper alignment and gentle core engagement in chair yoga contributes to improved posture, reducing strain on the spine.

7. Mind-Body Connection: The practice encourages a mindful connection between breath and movement, fostering a holistic approach to physical and mental well-being.

8. Social Interaction: Chair yoga classes provide a social setting, offering seniors an opportunity for interaction and a sense of community, which contributes to overall mental health.

9. Adaptability: Chair yoga is highly adaptable, accommodating individuals with different physical conditions and limitations, making it accessible to a broad audience.

10. Safe and Low-Impact: The practice is low-impact and conducted in a seated position, minimizing the risk of strain or injury, making it safe for seniors with various health concerns.

11. Increased Energy and Vitality: Regular participation in chair yoga can lead to increased energy levels, promoting a sense of vitality and overall improved quality of life.

12. Positive Mood and Emotional Well-Being: The combination of movement, breathwork, and relaxation fosters a positive

mood, contributing to emotional well-being and a more positive outlook on life.

13. Independence: Chair yoga supports seniors in maintaining independence by promoting functional mobility and providing tools to navigate daily activities with confidence.

14. Accessibility: The practice is accessible in various settings, including community centers, senior living facilities, or even at home, making it convenient for seniors to engage in regular physical activity.

1.4 Understanding Chair Yoga

Chair yoga aligns with the universal desire for wellness and stress relief. The practice's focus on holistic well-being, mindfulness, and relaxation resonates with people worldwide, transcending cultural differences.

Adaptability to Varied Lifestyles:

Chair yoga is highly adaptable, making it suitable for individuals with varying fitness levels, ages, and abilities.

Its versatility allows people with different cultural backgrounds to incorporate it into their lifestyles without significant modifications.

1.5 Origin and History of Chair Yoga

Chair yoga for seniors has its roots in traditional yoga practices but has been adapted to accommodate the specific needs and limitations of older individuals. The history of chair yoga involves a combination of ancient yoga principles and contemporary modifications to make the practice more accessible. Here's a summarized overview:

Ancient Yogic Principles:

The origins of chair yoga can be traced back to the ancient principles of yoga, which date back thousands of years in India. Traditional yoga encompasses a holistic approach to physical, mental, and spiritual well-being.

Integration of Props:

The concept of using props, including chairs, in yoga became more prominent in the 20th century. B.K.S. Iyengar, a renowned yoga teacher, emphasized the use of props to make yoga accessible to individuals with physical limitations.

Modern Adaptations:

As yoga gained popularity in the West, instructors began adapting traditional poses to cater to diverse populations, including seniors. The incorporation of chairs as a supportive prop became a key aspect of these adaptations.

Development for Seniors:

The specific development of chair yoga for seniors gained momentum in response to the growing aging population and the recognition of the unique challenges older individuals may face in traditional yoga settings.

Pioneering Instructors:

Pioneering yoga instructors, recognizing the benefits of yoga for seniors, started creating chair-based sequences and classes. This included modifying traditional poses and developing new techniques that could be comfortably performed while seated.

Promotion of Accessibility:

Chair yoga aligns with the broader movement in yoga to make the practice more inclusive and accessible to people of all ages and abilities. It addresses the diverse needs of seniors, including those with limited mobility, joint issues, or balance concerns.

Scientific Validation:

Over time, scientific studies have supported the efficacy of chair yoga for seniors in improving physical health, mental well-being, and overall quality of life. This validation has contributed to the continued growth and acceptance of chair yoga.

Integration into Wellness Programs:

Chair yoga has become a staple in wellness programs for seniors, often integrated into community centers, senior living facilities, and healthcare settings. It serves as a valuable tool for promoting active aging and maintaining health.

Global Adoption:s

Chair yoga's popularity has transcended cultural boundaries, and it is now practiced globally. Its adaptability and effectiveness have led to its incorporation into various health and wellness initiatives for seniors worldwide.

The digital age has facilitated the global dissemination of chair yoga through online platforms and resources.

Individuals worldwide can access chair yoga classes, tutorials, and information, breaking down geographical barriers and allowing for cross-cultural engagement.

Healthcare Recognition and Integration:

Recognition of chair yoga's therapeutic benefits by healthcare professionals has contributed to its integration into wellness programs globally.

Healthcare systems worldwide recommend chair yoga for its positive impact on physical and mental health, making it more widely accepted across cultures.

Cultural Sensitivity and Adaptations:

Chair yoga instructors and practitioners have demonstrated cultural sensitivity by incorporating adaptations that resonate with diverse audiences.

Cultural nuances, preferences, and traditional wellness practices are considered, making chair yoga more relatable and appealing to people from different cultural backgrounds.

Community Building and Inclusivity:

Chair yoga communities have embraced inclusivity, welcoming individuals from all walks of life.

Events, workshops, and classes promote diversity within the chair yoga community, fostering a sense of belonging that transcends cultural boundaries.

Integration into Workplace and Educational Settings:

The adaptability of chair yoga has led to its integration into workplace wellness programs and educational settings globally.

Employees and students from various cultural backgrounds find it accessible within their respective environments, contributing to its widespread acceptance.

Emphasis on Stress Reduction and Mindfulness:

The global appeal of stress reduction and mindfulness practices has propelled the popularity of chair yoga.

The practice's emphasis on mental well-being aligns with the universal need for stress relief, attracting individuals from different cultural contexts.

Cross-Cultural Training and Certification:

Chair yoga instructors and certification programs have recognized the importance of cross-cultural training.

Instructors are equipped to understand and address diverse cultural needs, making chair yoga more inclusive and culturally relevant.

Promotion of Testimonials and Success Stories:

The sharing of testimonials and success stories from individuals worldwide has played a crucial role in promoting chair yoga.

Real-life experiences create a global narrative that encourages others to explore chair yoga, irrespective of their cultural background.

Chair yoga's global popularity can be attributed to its universal appeal, adaptability, digital accessibility, healthcare recognition, cultural sensitivity, community inclusivity, workplace integration, stress reduction focus, cross-cultural training, and the promotion of personal stories that resonate across borders.

Regional adaptations in chair yoga practices may arise from cultural distinctions, traditional wellness methods, or specific considerations within particular communities. While chair yoga is inherently versatile, instructors and practitioners may introduce variations to align with local preferences or address distinct needs. Examples include integrating culturally specific breathing techniques, using traditional music or chants of significance, incorporating elements from traditional healing modalities, adjusting language and instructional style to suit regional preferences, discussing dietary habits in accordance with local cuisines, utilizing cultural symbolism in visualizations, emphasizing community and social aspects in regions where it holds importance, adapting practices to align with seasonal changes, and integrating principles from traditional medicine systems. These adaptations highlight chair yoga's ability to be flexible, catering to diverse cultural contexts while upholding its fundamental principles of accessibility and inclusivity.

Recent innovations and advancements in chair yoga techniques have been developed to cater specifically to the evolving needs of seniors, incorporating modern knowledge, research, and technology. Here are some noteworthy examples:

Technology Integration:

Online Classes and Apps: The use of online platforms and mobile applications has become prevalent, allowing seniors to access chair yoga classes from the comfort of their homes. This addresses the need for remote and flexible learning.

Virtual Reality (VR) Experiences:

Some chair yoga programs are exploring the integration of virtual reality experiences. Seniors can use VR headsets to engage in immersive and visually stimulating chair yoga sessions, enhancing the overall experience.

Smart Devices and Wearables:

The integration of smart devices and wearables allows seniors to track their movements, monitor vital signs, and receive personalized feedback during chair yoga sessions. This fosters a more interactive and tailored approach to their practice.

Adaptive Seating Solutions:

Innovations in adaptive seating solutions, such as ergonomic chairs with adjustable features, have been incorporated into chair yoga. These chairs provide better support and comfort, accommodating seniors with various physical needs.

Gamification of Chair Yoga:

Some chair yoga programs incorporate gamification elements to make the practice more engaging. This includes interactive challenges, rewards, and progress tracking, encouraging seniors to stay motivated and consistent in their practice.

Therapeutic Props and Equipment:

Specialized props and equipment, designed with seniors in mind, enhance the therapeutic aspects of chair yoga. This may include props that provide gentle resistance, support, or tactile stimulation, catering to different sensory needs.

Mindfulness and Meditation Apps:

Chair yoga programs often integrate mindfulness and meditation practices. Recent advancements include the development of user-friendly apps that guide seniors through meditation and relaxation exercises, promoting mental well-being.

Personalized Virtual Coaching:

Some chair yoga programs offer personalized virtual coaching sessions. Seniors can receive one-on-one guidance from certified instructors, addressing their specific health concerns and adapting the practice accordingly.

Inclusive Language and Instruction:

Innovations also extend to the inclusivity of language and instruction. There is a growing emphasis on using culturally sensitive and age-appropriate language to ensure that chair yoga is accessible and relatable to a diverse senior population.

Research-Backed Protocols:

Chair yoga advancements are increasingly informed by research on senior health. Evidence-based protocols are being developed to address specific health conditions, providing seniors with practices that are both safe and effective.

Intergenerational Programs:

Some chair yoga initiatives focus on intergenerational programs, bringing together seniors and younger generations. This fosters a sense of community and allows for the exchange of experiences and perspectives.

These recent innovations demonstrate the commitment to enhancing the chair yoga experience for seniors by leveraging technology, personalized approaches, and a deeper understanding of their evolving needs. The goal is to make chair yoga more engaging, accessible, and beneficial for the diverse senior population.

CHAPTER 2

Health Benefits of Chair Yoga

Chair yoga provides a variety of health advantages, serving as a gentle and accessible form of exercise, particularly beneficial for seniors or individuals with limited mobility. The detailed health benefits of chair yoga include:

2.1 Improved Flexibility:

Chair yoga involves gentle stretching exercises that enhance flexibility in muscles and joints, leading to increased range of motion for more comfortable daily activities.

Improved Joint Health:

The practice includes movements that promote joint health without imposing excessive stress, maintaining flexibility and reducing stiffness.

Seated poses in chair yoga target different muscle groups, fostering strength in the core, arms, legs, and back, supporting better posture and stability.

Balanced Stability:

Specific poses and exercises focus on improving balance and stability, crucial for preventing falls and maintaining independence, especially in the elderly.

Stress Reduction and Calmness:

Mindful breathing and relaxation techniques integrated into chair yoga contribute to stress reduction, activating the parasympathetic nervous system for a sense of calm.

Posture Improvement:

Chair yoga emphasizes body alignment awareness and encourages proper posture, alleviating back and neck pain associated with poor alignment.

Enhanced Circulation:

Gentle movements and controlled breathing support improved blood circulation, benefiting cardiovascular health and overall oxygenation of tissues.

Mind-Body Harmony:

Chair yoga cultivates a connection between the mind and body through mindful movements and breath awareness, enhancing mental focus and cognitive function.

Pain Management:

Adaptations for chronic pain conditions in chair yoga offer gentle movements to ease discomfort, potentially reducing the need for pain medications.

Respiratory Function Improvement:

Respiratory function improvement in chair yoga for seniors is a key focus aimed at enhancing lung capacity, promoting efficient breathing, and contributing to overall respiratory health. The practice incorporates tailored exercises to address the specific needs and limitations of older individuals. Here's a summarized overview:

Diaphragmatic Breathing:

- Chair yoga emphasizes diaphragmatic breathing, also known as belly breathing. This technique encourages seniors to engage the diaphragm fully, promoting deeper breaths and increased oxygen intake.

Lung Capacity Expansion:

- Specific chair yoga poses and breathing exercises are designed to expand lung capacity gradually. These exercises work to open up the chest and improve the ability of the lungs to take in and release air.

Slow and Controlled Breathing:

- Seniors are guided to practice slow and controlled breathing patterns during chair yoga. This deliberate approach helps enhance respiratory function, reduce breathlessness, and promote relaxation.

Incorporation of Pranayama:

- Pranayama, or breath control techniques, are integrated into chair yoga sessions. Techniques like paced breathing and alternate nostril breathing are adapted to the seated position, supporting respiratory well-being.

Ribcage Mobility Exercises:

- Chair yoga includes exercises that focus on mobilizing the ribcage. These movements enhance the flexibility of the chest and rib muscles, facilitating improved respiratory function.

Mindful Breath Awareness:

- Mindfulness is incorporated into the practice, encouraging seniors to maintain awareness of their breath. This mindfulness promotes a connection between breath and movement, contributing to improved respiratory function.

Breath Retention Practices:

- Gentle breath retention practices, such as inhale and hold or exhale and hold, may be introduced. These exercises help strengthen respiratory muscles and enhance breath control.

Posture Alignment for Optimal Breathing:

- Emphasis is placed on maintaining proper posture during chair yoga, ensuring optimal alignment for effective breathing. Correct posture supports the natural expansion and contraction of the lungs.

Integration of Relaxation Techniques:

- Chair yoga incorporates relaxation techniques to reduce tension in respiratory muscles. This relaxation contributes to improved breathing patterns and overall respiratory function.

Adapted Prone and Supine Poses:

- Certain prone and supine poses may be adapted to the seated position, allowing seniors to experience the benefits of poses that traditionally enhance lung capacity and respiratory function.

Breath Coordination with Movement:

- Movement sequences in chair yoga are coordinated with breath patterns. Seniors learn to synchronize their breath with gentle movements, promoting efficient and rhythmic breathing.

Gradual Progression:

- Chair yoga sessions are designed with a focus on gradual progression. This approach allows seniors to build respiratory strength and function at their own pace, considering individual capabilities.

Boosted Energy Levels:

Chair yoga's combination of movements, stretching, and mindful breathing can boost energy levels, leaving participants feeling more invigorated and alert.

Emotional Well-Being:

Elements like mindfulness and meditation positively impact emotional well-being, contributing to stress reduction and emotional balance.

Social Connection:

Chair yoga classes provide a supportive and social environment, fostering connections among participants and contributing to a sense of community.

Enhancing balance and stability in chair yoga for seniors involves incorporating specific exercises and modifications to support the unique needs of older individuals. The primary focus is on promoting physical stability, preventing falls, and improving overall well-being. Key elements of chair yoga for seniors include:

Seated Poses: Most exercises are performed while sitting in a chair, ensuring comfort and accessibility. Seated poses help seniors build strength, flexibility, and balance without putting undue stress on joints.

Breathing Techniques: Mindful breathing is integrated to enhance concentration and relaxation. Controlled breathing not only improves lung capacity but also contributes to mental focus and stress reduction.

Gentle Stretching: Chair yoga incorporates gentle stretches to improve flexibility and joint mobility. These stretches are designed to be safe for seniors, promoting increased range of motion.

Core Strengthening: Emphasis is placed on strengthening the core muscles to enhance overall stability. This is particularly important for seniors to support their posture and prevent falls.

Adaptations for Limited Mobility: Chair yoga can be adapted for individuals with limited mobility or specific health concerns. Modifications are made to accommodate seniors with various physical conditions.

Mind-Body Connection: The practice encourages a mind-body connection, fostering a sense of awareness and mindfulness. This can contribute to improved mental well-being and reduced stress.

Gradual Progression: The program typically involves a gradual progression of difficulty to accommodate seniors of varying fitness levels. This allows participants to work at their own pace and gradually build strength and stability.

Joint health and mobility in yoga for seniors are essential components that focus on maintaining and improving the flexibility, strength, and overall well-being of the joints. The approach is adapted to suit the unique needs and considerations of older individuals. Here's a summarized overview:

Gentle Joint Movements:

Yoga for seniors incorporates gentle movements that target various joints, promoting flexibility without placing excessive strain. These movements include rotations, circles, and controlled stretches.

Focus on Major Joints:

Emphasis is placed on major joints such as the knees, hips, shoulders, and spine. Poses and exercises are designed to enhance the range of motion in these key areas, addressing common issues associated with aging.

Dynamic Stretching:

Dynamic stretching exercises are included to encourage joints to move through their full range, helping to improve flexibility and reduce stiffness. These controlled movements are performed with mindful awareness.

Seated and Supported Poses:

Many yoga poses are modified to a seated position, allowing seniors to engage in joint-friendly movements comfortably. Support from chairs or props is often incorporated to ensure stability.

Balanced Approach:

Yoga sequences for seniors strike a balance between providing gentle challenges to joints and ensuring safety. The intention is to improve mobility without causing stress or discomfort.

Weight-Bearing Poses:

Weight-bearing poses, adapted to accommodate individual capabilities, are integrated into the practice. These poses contribute to joint strength and bone density.

Joint Stabilization Exercises:

Yoga for seniors includes exercises that promote joint stabilization. This helps enhance the overall integrity of the joints and supports seniors in maintaining balance and coordination.

Breath Awareness:

Mindful breathing techniques are incorporated to promote relaxation and reduce tension around joints. This mindful approach enhances the mind-body connection and contributes to joint health.

Adaptability and Modifications:

Instructors emphasize the adaptability of poses to suit individual needs. Modifications are encouraged based on participants' joint health, ensuring that the practice is accessible and safe for all.

Prop Utilization:

Warm-Up and Cool Down:

Yoga sessions for seniors include thorough warm-up and cool-down periods. The warm-up prepares joints for movement, while the cool-down incorporates gentle stretches to promote relaxation and flexibility.

Hydration Emphasis:

Hydration is emphasized to support joint health. Staying adequately hydrated contributes to the lubrication of joints and helps prevent stiffness and discomfort.

2.3 Stress Reduction and Mental Well-being:

Mindful Breathing Techniques:

Chair yoga for seniors emphasizes mindful breathing, including deep belly breathing and conscious inhalation and exhalation. These techniques aim to reduce stress and enhance awareness of the breath.

Gentle Movement and Stretching:

The practice incorporates gentle movements and stretches that can be comfortably done while seated. These movements promote relaxation, improve flexibility, and contribute to a sense of well-being.

Guided Imagery and Visualization:

Guided imagery encourages seniors to visualize calming scenes or engage in positive visualizations. This technique serves as a mental escape and contributes to mental well-being.

Progressive Muscle Relaxation:

Techniques like progressive muscle relaxation are integrated, guiding seniors to consciously tense and release different muscle groups. This practice helps release physical tension and induce relaxation.

Meditation and Mindfulness:

Chair yoga sessions include meditation practices, fostering mindfulness to cultivate a focused and present state of mind. Seniors learn to observe thoughts without judgment, promoting mental clarity and calmness.

Yoga Nidra (Yogic Sleep):

The practice may include Yoga Nidra, a guided relaxation technique that promotes conscious rest and stress reduction, contributing to overall mental well-being.

Positive Affirmations:

Encouraging the use of positive affirmations during chair yoga enhances a positive mindset. Seniors are guided to cultivate self-compassion and affirmations that contribute to mental well-being.

Social Interaction:

Group chair yoga sessions provide a social setting, fostering a sense of community and support. Social interaction plays a role in reducing feelings of isolation and positively impacting mental health.

Soothing Music and Sounds:

The use of soothing music or nature sounds enhances the calming atmosphere during chair yoga sessions. Auditory components contribute to stress reduction and mental relaxation.

Stress-Relief Breathing Techniques:

Specific breathing techniques designed for stress relief, such as extended exhalation or 4-7-8 breathing, are incorporated. These techniques activate the body's relaxation response.

Cognitive Focus:

Mindful attention redirects cognitive focus away from stressors. Seniors are guided to immerse themselves in the present moment, promoting a break from worrisome thoughts.

Adapted Relaxation Poses:

Chair yoga sessions conclude with adapted relaxation poses that allow seniors to unwind and release tension. These poses contribute to an overall sense of tranquility and mental well-being.

CHAPTER 3

GETTING STARTED WITH CHAIR YOGA

3.1 Safety Considerations

Commencing chair yoga for seniors involves establishing a safe and tailored environment to accommodate the unique needs of older individuals. Here's an overview of essential steps:

Participant Assessment:

Evaluate the health, mobility, and any physical constraints of participants before initiating chair yoga to customize the practice accordingly.

Appropriate Seating Selection:

Choose stable chairs with flat seats, devoid of wheels, and place them on a non-slip surface to prevent accidents.

Gentle Warm-up:

Begin with a mild warm-up to prepare the body, including seated neck stretches, shoulder rolls, and ankle circles.

Basic Breathing Exercises:

Integrate simple breathing exercises to encourage relaxation and mindfulness, emphasizing slow, deep breaths.

Seated Poses:

Introduce seated yoga poses, modified to accommodate chairs, focusing on enhancing strength, flexibility, and balance.

Posture Guidance:

Emphasize proper posture, instructing participants to sit upright, engage core muscles, and relax shoulders.

Adaptations and Props:

Utilize props like blocks or cushions for support, adapting poses based on individual abilities and needs.

Mindfulness and Relaxation:

Include mindfulness and relaxation techniques, such as guided imagery or meditation, to promote relaxation.

Gradual Progression:

Structure sessions to allow a gradual increase in difficulty, starting with basic poses and introducing more challenging movements over time.

Encourage Social Interaction:

Foster a sense of community during chair yoga sessions, creating a supportive and enjoyable atmosphere for seniors.

Regular Check-ins:

Conduct periodic check-ins with participants to assess their experience, address concerns, and gather feedback for program refinement.

Creating a comfortable space for yoga sessions tailored to seniors involves thoughtful considerations to address their unique needs and enhance the overall experience. Here's a summary of key aspects:

Accessible Seating:

Choose stable and supportive chairs with flat seats, ensuring they are free of wheels and placed on a non-slip surface to prevent accidents.

Adequate Lighting:

Ensure the space is well-lit to promote visibility and a sense of security, minimizing the risk of tripping or discomfort during the practice.

Ample Ventilation:

Maintain good air circulation to ensure a comfortable and refreshing atmosphere, enhancing the overall well-being of participants.

Quiet and Calm Environment:

Minimize external noise and distractions to create a serene and focused setting, allowing seniors to fully engage in the yoga practice.

Clear Pathways:

Remove any potential obstacles or clutter to provide seniors with clear and safe pathways, facilitating easy movement during the session.

Temperature Control:

Maintain a comfortable room temperature, considering that seniors may be more sensitive to extremes of heat or cold. This ensures a pleasant and adaptable environment.

Non-Slip Flooring:

Choose flooring that is non-slip to prevent accidents, especially during movements or transitions between poses. This is crucial for the safety of participants.

Personal Space Consideration:

Arrange participants' chairs with enough space between them to allow for comfortable and unobstructed movement during the yoga practice.

Mindful Decor:

Consider incorporating calming elements such as soothing colors, plants, or gentle artwork to contribute to a tranquil and inviting atmosphere.

Seating Arrangement:

Arrange the chairs in a circular or semi-circle formation to create a sense of inclusivity and facilitate interaction among participants.

Participant Feedback:

Encourage feedback from participants regarding the comfort of the space, allowing for adjustments and improvements based on their preferences and needs.

By implementing these considerations, the setup for yoga sessions for seniors can be optimized for comfort, safety, and an overall positive experience tailored to their well-being.

3.3. Basic Equipment and Props

In yoga for seniors, the use of basic equipment and props plays a crucial role in providing support, enhancing comfort, and accommodating varying levels of mobility. Here's an overview of essential equipment and props commonly used in senior yoga sessions:

Yoga Mats:

Provide non-slip yoga mats to create a comfortable and stable foundation for seated and standing poses. Mats offer support and prevent slips, enhancing safety during the practice.

Sturdy Chairs:

Use stable and supportive chairs with flat seats for seated poses. Chairs with no wheels and a firm structure provide a secure base for seniors to practice without the risk of instability.

Blocks:

Yoga blocks are useful for modifying poses and providing additional height or support. They can be placed under the hands, feet, or hips to make certain poses more accessible and comfortable.

Straps:

Yoga straps help seniors achieve proper alignment in poses by extending their reach. They are particularly beneficial for individuals with limited flexibility or range of motion.

Cushions and Bolsters:

Provide cushions or bolsters to enhance comfort during seated poses and relaxation at the end of the session. These props can be used to support the lower back or provide extra padding as needed.

Blankets:

Blankets offer warmth and padding during relaxation poses and can also be used for support under joints or sensitive areas. They add an extra layer of comfort for seniors.

Eye Pillows:

Eye pillows can be used during relaxation or meditation to block out light and create a soothing environment, promoting a deeper sense of calm and relaxation.

Therabands or Resistance Bands:

These elastic bands can be incorporated into the practice to add gentle resistance for strength-building exercises, contributing to improved muscle tone and flexibility.

Gentle Exercise Balls:

Soft and pliable exercise balls can be used for various exercises to enhance balance, stability, and core strength while providing a comfortable surface for the hands or other body parts.

Stability Discs: These inflatable discs can be placed on chairs or the floor to add an element of instability, challenging participants' balance and engaging core muscles in a controlled manner.

Foot Rollers:

Designed to massage and stimulate the feet, foot rollers can be beneficial for seniors, especially those dealing with foot-related issues or seeking additional foot comfort.

Adaptive Props:

Consider other adaptive props based on individual needs, such as yoga wedges, which can assist in modifying poses to accommodate specific physical conditions.

By incorporating these basic equipment and props, yoga for seniors becomes a more accessible, comfortable, and adaptable practice, promoting a positive and inclusive experience for participants.

4.1. Breathing Techniques for Relaxation

Breathing techniques for relaxation in chair yoga for seniors play a central role in promoting a calm and mindful practice. These techniques are tailored to enhance relaxation, reduce stress, and improve overall well-being. Key aspects of incorporating breathing techniques during chair yoga for seniors include:

Mindful Breathing Focus:

Participants are guided to bring attention to their breath, emphasizing slow, deep inhalations and exhalations. Mindful breathing serves as a focal point to enhance relaxation and mental presence.

Diaphragmatic Breathing:

Emphasis is placed on diaphragmatic breathing, where seniors are encouraged to breathe deeply into their diaphragm rather than shallow chest breathing. This technique promotes a more relaxed and efficient breath pattern.

Extended Exhalation:

Incorporating a longer exhalation helps activate the body's relaxation response. Seniors are guided to extend the duration of their exhales, fostering a sense of calm and stress reduction.

Counted Breathing:

Counting breaths provides a structured approach to breathing exercises. This can involve inhaling for a specific count, holding the breath briefly, and then exhaling for an equal count, promoting rhythmic and controlled breathing.

Alternate Nostril Breathing:

The practice of alternate nostril breathing, or Nadi Shodhana, is introduced. This technique involves breathing in and out through one nostril at a time, promoting balance and relaxation.

4-7-8 Breathing:

The 4-7-8 breathing technique is incorporated, where seniors inhale for a count of four, hold the breath for a count of seven, and exhale for a count of eight. This pattern is repeated to induce a sense of calmness.

Guided Imagery Breathing:

Breathing is combined with guided imagery, encouraging seniors to visualize calming scenes or sensations. This enhances relaxation and creates a positive mental space.

Coordinated Movement and Breath:

Breath awareness is synchronized with gentle movements, such as raising and lowering arms. This coordination fosters a mind-body connection, enhancing relaxation and concentration.

Relaxing Breath Pacing:

Encourage a relaxed pacing of breath throughout the session, avoiding rushed or forced breathing. This approach supports a soothing and comfortable experience.

Closing Relaxation Breath:

The session concludes with a period of intentional relaxation breathing, allowing seniors to unwind, release tension, and experience the calming effects of controlled breathwork.

4.2 Warm-up Exercises for Joints and Muscles

Focus on hip circles, knee lifts, and gentle leg swings to warm up the lower body and increase joint mobility.

Ankle and Foot Warm-up:

Ankle circles and toe-pointing exercises help improve circulation and flexibility in the lower extremities.

Breathing Exercises:

Include mindful breathing exercises to center the mind, increase lung capacity, and promote relaxation.

Mindful Movement:

Encourage slow, controlled movements with an emphasis on mindfulness to connect the body and mind.

Adaptations and Modifications:

Provide variations and modifications for each exercise to accommodate individual abilities and limitations.

Safety First:

Emphasize the importance of listening to the body, avoiding pain, and moving within a comfortable range to ensure a safe practice.

In yoga for seniors, the warm-up is designed to be gentle, accessible, and adapted to the unique needs of older individuals. It aims to create a supportive environment for seniors to enhance flexibility, improve joint function, and promote overall well-being. Always encourage seniors to work at their own pace, respecting their bodies and limitations while enjoying the benefits of yoga practice.

4.3 Guided chair yoga sessions for seniors

They are thoughtfully designed practices that cater to the unique needs and capabilities of older individuals. These sessions offer a gentle and accessible approach to yoga, emphasizing seated postures, breathing exercises, and mindful movements. Here's a detailed and comprehensive explanation of the key elements involved in guided chair yoga sessions:

1. Seated Postures and Movements:

Purpose: The primary focus is on seated postures and movements to accommodate seniors, allowing them to engage in the practice comfortably without the need for standing or complex poses.

Implementation: Participants perform a variety of yoga poses adapted to the seated position, promoting flexibility, strength, and balance.

2. Breath-Centered Practices:

Purpose: Guided chair yoga places a strong emphasis on breath-centered practices to improve respiratory function, reduce stress, and enhance relaxation.

Implementation: Participants engage in diaphragmatic breathing, deep inhalations, and exhalations, fostering a connection between breath and movement.

3. Gentle Warm-Up:

Purpose: A gentle warm-up is incorporated to prepare the body for the session, increase blood flow, and promote flexibility.

Implementation: Warm-up activities include neck and shoulder rolls, wrist stretches, and subtle movements designed to awaken the body gradually.

4. Joint Mobility Exercises:

Purpose: To improve joint flexibility and mobility, focusing on major joints such as wrists, ankles, hips, and shoulders.

Implementation: Participants engage in gentle joint rotations, circles, and controlled stretches, promoting overall joint health.

5. Adapted Asanas (Poses):

Purpose: Traditional yoga poses are adapted to the seated position, ensuring that seniors experience the benefits of each pose safely and comfortably.

Implementation: Poses may include modified versions of seated forward bends, twists, and gentle backbends, with the chair providing support.

6. Mindful Stretching:

Purpose: To encourage mindful awareness of the body, fostering a deeper connection between breath and movement.

Implementation: Participants engage in stretches with focused attention, allowing them to be present in the moment and cultivate body awareness.

7. Balance Enhancement Techniques:

Purpose: To improve stability, coordination, and prevent falls by incorporating balance-enhancing exercises.

Implementation: Seated balancing poses and movements challenge participants in a controlled and safe manner, enhancing overall stability.

8. Relaxation and Meditation:

Purpose: Guided chair yoga includes practices that promote relaxation and meditation, reducing stress and fostering mental well-being.

Implementation: Sessions often end with guided relaxation techniques, meditation, or a brief period of seated mindfulness.

9. Incorporation of Props:

Purpose: To enhance comfort and support during poses, accommodating individual needs.

Implementation: Props such as blocks, straps, or cushions may be used to assist in poses and ensure that the practice is adaptable to individual requirements.

10. Progressive Movement Sequencing:

Purpose: A gradual progression of movements allows participants to build strength, flexibility, and confidence over time.

Implementation: Sequences are carefully structured, encouraging participants to advance at their own pace while enjoying the benefits of a progressive practice.

11. Encouraging Social Engagement:

Purpose: Group dynamics create a supportive community atmosphere, fostering social interaction and a sense of shared experience.

Implementation: Participants engage in chair yoga within a group setting, providing encouragement, camaraderie, and mutual support.

12. Cool-Down Ritual and Serene Closure:

Purpose: To bring the body to a state of relaxation and provide a peaceful closure to the session.

Implementation: Cool-down activities include gentle stretches, and the session may conclude with a brief seated meditation or relaxation pose, allowing participants to absorb the benefits of the Chair Yoga Sessions.

CHAPTER 5

Building Flexibility and Strength

5.1 Progressive Chair Yoga Poses

Progressive chair yoga poses for seniors are designed to gradually enhance flexibility, strength, and balance in a safe and accessible manner. These poses are adapted to the seated position, accommodating the unique needs of older individuals. Key features of progressive chair yoga poses for seniors include:

Seated Mountain Pose:

Seniors start in a seated position with a focus on alignment, engaging core muscles, and reaching arms overhead. This foundational pose promotes posture and balance.

Seated Forward Bend:

Participants gently hinge at the hips while seated, reaching towards their toes. This pose promotes flexibility in the spine, stretches the hamstrings, and encourages relaxation.

Seated Twist:

Seniors rotate their upper body while seated, promoting spinal flexibility and mobility. This twist engages the core and contributes to a sense of well-being.

Seated Cat-Cow Stretch:

Participants perform a modified cat-cow stretch while seated, arching and rounding the spine. This movement enhances flexibility and mobility in the spine.

Chair Warrior Poses:

Modified versions of warrior poses are adapted for the chair, promoting leg strength, stability, and gentle hip opening.

Seated Hip Opener:

This pose involves gently opening the hips while seated, promoting flexibility and relieving tension in the hip joints.

Chair Pigeon Pose:

Seniors perform a seated version of the pigeon pose, stretching the outer hips and promoting flexibility. This pose is beneficial for those with tight hips.

Seated Leg Lifts:

Participants lift one leg at a time while seated, targeting the quadriceps and hip flexors. This exercise helps build strength in the lower body.

Seated Side Stretch:

Seniors perform gentle stretches to the sides while seated, promoting flexibility in the torso and stretching the muscles along the sides of the body.

Seated Tree Pose:

This modified version of the tree pose is performed while seated, focusing on balance and stability. It involves placing one foot on the inner thigh of the opposite leg.

Chair Downward-Facing Dog:

Participants place their hands on the back of the chair, creating a modified downward-facing dog position. This pose stretches the spine, shoulders, and hamstrings.

Seated Relaxation Pose:

The session concludes with a seated relaxation pose, allowing seniors to focus on deep, controlled breathing and experience a sense of calm and tranquility.

5.2 Incorporating resistance and stretching

Incorporating resistance and stretching in yoga for seniors involves a balanced approach to enhance strength, flexibility, and overall well-being. This tailored practice aims to provide gentle yet effective exercises, taking into consideration the unique needs and limitations of older individuals. Key aspects of incorporating resistance and stretching in yoga for seniors include:

Gentle Resistance Training:

Utilize resistance bands or light weights to introduce gentle resistance into the yoga routine. This helps seniors build muscle strength gradually, particularly focusing on areas like the arms, shoulders, and legs.

Functional Movements:

Integrate functional movements that mimic daily activities, promoting strength and mobility. This approach enhances overall functionality and supports seniors in their day-to-day tasks.

Balancing Resistance:

Emphasize exercises that incorporate balance while using resistance. This can include leg lifts or arm movements that challenge stability, promoting improved balance and coordination.

Dynamic Stretching:

Incorporate dynamic stretching, involving controlled movements that take joints through their full range of motion. This helps improve flexibility, joint mobility, and circulation.

Static Stretching:

Include static stretching exercises to elongate muscles and improve flexibility. Holding stretches for a moderate duration aids in reducing muscle tension and promoting relaxation.

Focus on Major Muscle Groups:

Design exercises that target major muscle groups, such as the quadriceps, hamstrings, chest, and back. This comprehensive approach ensures a balanced and effective workout.

Joint-Friendly Stretching:

Modify traditional yoga poses to make them joint-friendly, ensuring that stretching exercises are gentle and accessible for seniors. Props like blocks or cushions can be used for additional support.

Breath-Centric Stretching:

Encourage seniors to synchronize their breath with stretching movements. This mindful approach enhances relaxation and fosters a mind-body connection during the practice.

Adaptability and Progression:

Allow for adaptability in resistance and stretching exercises to accommodate varying fitness levels and individual capabilities. Gradual progression ensures that seniors can comfortably improve their strength and flexibility over time.

Warm-Up and Cool Down:

Begin sessions with a gentle warm-up to prepare the body for movement, incorporating light cardio and joint mobility exercises. Conclude with a cool-down that includes static stretches to promote flexibility and relaxation.

Guided Instruction:

Provide clear and guided instructions, emphasizing proper form and alignment during resistance and stretching exercises. This helps prevent injuries and ensures a safe and effective practice.

Participant Feedback:

Encourage participants to provide feedback on their comfort levels and any physical limitations. This information helps tailor the resistance and stretching routine to individual needs.

5.3 Strategies for Seniors with Limited Mobility

Modify the chair itself, considering adjustments such as adding cushions or using chairs with different seat heights to accommodate diverse mobility levels and physical conditions.

Adapted Breathing Techniques:

Emphasize breathing techniques suitable for a seated position, such as deep belly breathing, mindful breath awareness, and gentle pranayama exercises.

Gentle Movement Sequences:

Design slow and controlled movement sequences targeting various body areas, fostering improved mobility through gradual and mindful motions.

Focus on Range of Motion:

Prioritize poses that enhance joint range of motion, incorporating gentle circular motions for wrists, ankles, and shoulders.

Seated Meditation:

Integrate seated meditation or mindfulness practices to allow seniors to focus on mental well-being while remaining comfortably seated, promoting relaxation and stress reduction.

Encourage Individual Pace:

Stress the importance of participants engaging in the practice at their own pace, listening to their bodies, and only proceeding as far as they feel comfortable.

Offer Options and Alternatives:

Provide variations for poses and exercises, ensuring that seniors with varying mobility levels can choose options that suit their abilities and comfort.

Include Chair Support:

Use the chair as a supportive prop in poses, such as incorporating seated forward bends where participants can use the chair for arm support.

Water Breaks and Rest Periods:

Schedule breaks and rest periods, allowing seniors to hydrate and rest as needed, ensuring that the practice remains enjoyable and manageable.

Educate on Benefits:

Share information on the positive impacts of chair yoga, highlighting how the practice can enhance circulation, reduce stiffness, and contribute to overall well-being for seniors with limited mobility.

CHAPTER 6

6.1 Importance of Balance for Seniors

Balance is a fundamental aspect of well-being, particularly for seniors who may face challenges related to mobility and stability. This chapter explores the critical importance of balance for seniors in the context of chair yoga. It delves into the significance of balance, the specific considerations for seniors, and how chair yoga can play a pivotal role in enhancing and maintaining balance.

Understanding the Significance of Balance:

Maintaining Independence:

Balance is essential for daily activities, allowing seniors to maintain independence. A strong sense of balance contributes to the ability to walk, stand, and perform routine tasks without assistance.

Fall Prevention:

Balance is closely linked to fall prevention. Seniors with compromised balance are at a higher risk of falls, which can have severe consequences. Strengthening balance can significantly reduce this risk.

Overall Physical Well-being:

A well-balanced body contributes to overall physical well-being. It supports proper posture, reduces muscle imbalances, and minimizes the strain on joints, promoting longevity and vitality.

Challenges to Balance in Seniors:

Age-Related Changes:

Seniors experience natural age-related changes, including a decline in muscle mass, joint flexibility, and proprioception, all of which can affect balance.

Medical Conditions:

Certain medical conditions, medications, and sensory impairments can further challenge balance in seniors. Conditions such as arthritis, vestibular issues, or neuropathy may impact stability.

Role of Chair Yoga in Balancing for Seniors:

Seated Balance Poses:

Chair yoga introduces a range of seated balance poses that target the core and lower body muscles. These poses help seniors build strength and stability while providing support through the chair.

Adapted Standing Poses:

Chair yoga can incorporate adapted standing poses with the chair as a supportive prop. This allows seniors to work on balance while having the security of the chair within reach.

Proprioception Enhancement:

Chair yoga emphasizes mindful movements, enhancing proprioception—the awareness of one's body in space. This heightened awareness contributes to improved balance and coordination. Core Strengthening:

Core strength is crucial for balance. Chair yoga includes exercises that target the core muscles, promoting stability and reducing the risk of falls.

Gradual Progression:

Chair yoga sessions are designed to gradually progress in difficulty, allowing seniors to build balance at their own pace. This approach ensures that participants can safely advance their abilities over time.

Benefits of Improved Balance:

Increased Confidence:

As seniors experience improved balance through chair yoga, their confidence in performing daily activities and engaging in physical movement grows.

Enhanced Mobility:

Better balance positively impacts overall mobility. Seniors with improved balance can move more freely, which is essential for maintaining an active and independent lifestyle.

Joint Balanced movement in chair yoga helps maintain joint health. It reduces the risk of overloading joints and minimizes the impact on areas prone to age-related stiffness.

Incorporating Balance into Chair Yoga Sessions:

Mindful Movement:

Chair yoga emphasizes mindful movement, encouraging seniors to be present and focused. This awareness enhances balance by fostering a connection between the body and the mind.

Breath Coordination:

Coordination of breath with movement in chair yoga contributes to balance. Breath awareness promotes concentration and helps participants stay centered during poses.

Modifications and Support:

Instructors provide modifications and support, ensuring that participants can safely engage in balance-focused poses. The use of props, including the chair, adds an element of security.

Progressive Sequencing:

Chair yoga sessions follow a progressive sequencing of poses, introducing balance-focused exercises gradually. This approach allows seniors to build strength and stability over time.

Balance is a crucial aspect of overall well-being, particularly for seniors. Chair yoga offers a gentle and supportive way for older individuals to enhance their balance. This subchapter explores a selection of chair yoga poses specifically designed to improve balance, promoting stability and reducing the risk of falls.

1. Seated Mountain Pose:

Purpose: Grounding and centering pose to improve posture and overall body awareness.

Execution:

Sit comfortably on the chair with feet flat on the floor.

Engage the core and lengthen the spine.

Inhale, raising arms overhead with palms facing each other.

Exhale, bringing hands to heart center.

2. Chair Warrior I:

Purpose: Strengthens legs and core, enhancing stability.

Execution:

Sit forward on the chair, extend one leg back.

Keep the front knee bent at a 90-degree angle.

Inhale, raising arms overhead.

Hold for a few breaths and switch sides.

3. Seated Tree Pose:

Purpose: Enhances balance and focus while seated.

Execution:

Sit with a tall spine, feet flat on the floor.

Lift one foot and place the sole against the inner thigh or calf.

Find a focal point and bring hands to heart center.

4. Leg Lifts:

Purpose: Strengthens leg muscles and improves balance.

Execution:

Sit tall, extend one leg forward.

Hold for a few breaths and lower.

Repeat on the other leg, gradually increasing repetitions.

5. Chair Cat-Cow Stretch:

Purpose: Promotes flexibility and balance in the spine.

Execution:

Sit forward on the chair, hands on knees.

Inhale, arching the back (Cow Pose).

Exhale, rounding the spine (Cat Pose).

6. Seated Twist:

Purpose: Enhances spinal mobility and balance.

Execution:

Sit tall, place one hand on the opposite knee.

Inhale, lengthen the spine; exhale, twist gently.

Hold for a few breaths, switch sides.

7. Chair Squats:

Purpose: Strengthens lower body muscles and improves stability.

Execution:

Stand in front of the chair with feet hip-width apart.

Inhale, lowering into a squat, keeping knees over ankles.

Exhale, return to a standing position.

8. Seated Side Stretch:

Purpose: Stretches the side body and improves balance.

Execution:

Sit tall, reach one arm overhead, leaning to the opposite side.

Feel the stretch along the side of the body.

Hold for a few breaths, switch sides.

9. Chair Balance Pose:

Purpose: Challenges balance and stability.

Execution:

Sit forward on the chair, lift one foot a few inches off the floor.

Hold onto the chair for support.

Gradually increase the hold time and switch legs.

10. Seated Forward Bend:

Purpose: Stretches the spine and improves balance.

Execution:

Sit forward on the chair with feet flat.

Inhale, lengthen the spine; exhale, hinge at the hips and reach forward.

11. Chair Warrior II:

Purpose: Strengthens legs and improves balance in a seated position.

Execution:

Sit on the chair with feet wide apart.

Turn one foot outward, bend the knee, and extend arms parallel to the floor.

Hold for a few breaths and switch sides.

12. Seated Knee Lifts:

Purpose: Strengthens abdominal muscles and improves balance.

Execution:

Sit tall, lift one knee toward the chest.

Hold for a few breaths and lower.

Repeat on the other leg.

6.3 Gradual Progression and Modifications

Balance and safety are paramount in chair yoga for seniors. This subchapter delves into the significance of gradual progression and modifications, providing a detailed exploration of how these principles can be implemented to ensure a safe and effective practice.

 Understanding the Importance of Gradual Progression:

1 Adapting to Individual Needs:

Gradual progression acknowledges the diverse abilities and limitations of seniors. It allows participants to adapt the practice to their own pace, fostering a sense of achievement without overexertion.

2 Building Strength and Confidence:

Progressing gradually helps seniors build strength and confidence over time. This approach ensures that each stage of the practice is manageable and contributes positively to physical well-being.

Starting with Foundation Poses:

Begin with foundational poses that are easily accessible. Focus on seated postures that establish a connection between breath and movement, allowing seniors to become comfortable with the basic principles of chair yoga.

Incremental Time and Intensity:

Gradually increase the duration and intensity of poses. For instance, start with shorter holding times and minimal repetitions, gradually progressing to longer durations and more challenging variations as participants gain strength and confidence.

Introducing Supported Standing Poses:

As participants become more accustomed to seated poses, introduce supported standing poses with the chair as a stabilizing prop. This progression enhances balance and strength in a gradual and secure manner.

Incorporating Gentle Transitions:

Encourage gentle transitions between poses. Smooth transitions enhance fluidity and help seniors adapt to changes in movement patterns, promoting a sense of ease and comfort in the practice.

Poses to Individual Abilities:

Modifications in chair yoga involve adapting poses to accommodate the unique abilities of each participant. This ensures that individuals with varying levels of flexibility, strength, or mobility can engage comfortably.

Variations for Different Levels:

Offer variations for poses to cater to different proficiency levels. Providing options allows seniors to choose the modification that suits their comfort level, empowering them to tailor the practice to their capabilities.

Encouraging Communication:

Foster open communication between instructors and participants. Encourage seniors to share any discomfort or concerns, allowing for immediate modifications or adjustments to ensure a safe and enjoyable experience.

Implementing Gradual Progression and Modifications in Sample Sequences:

Sample Sequence for Beginners:

Start with seated warm-up exercises, gradually introducing simple seated poses like Seated Mountain Pose and Seated Tree Pose. Progress to gentle standing poses with the chair for support, such as Supported Standing Forward Bend.

Intermediate Sample Sequence:

Include a mix of seated and standing poses with a focus on balance, such as Chair Warrior I and Chair Warrior II. Incorporate gentle transitions and encourage participants to explore variations that suit their comfort level.

Advanced Sample Sequence:

For more advanced participants, incorporate challenging seated and standing poses like Seated Twist and Chair Balance Pose. Emphasize smooth transitions and longer holding times to further enhance strength and stability.

CHAPTER 7

Integrating Chair Yoga into Daily Life

7.1 Creating a Consistent Practice

Consistency is key in deriving the maximum benefits from chair yoga for seniors. This subchapter explores the elements involved in establishing and maintaining a regular and meaningful chair yoga practice, considering factors such as motivation, scheduling, and adapting the practice to individual needs.

Understanding the Importance of Consistency:

1 Building Muscle Memory:

Regular practice helps seniors build muscle memory, enhancing their ability to perform poses with greater ease and fluidity over time.

2 Incremental Progress:

Consistency allows for incremental progress. Seniors can gradually improve flexibility, strength, and balance by incorporating chair yoga into their routine consistently.

3 Mental and Emotional Benefits:

A consistent chair yoga practice contributes to mental and emotional well-being. The meditative aspects of the practice can reduce stress, promote relaxation, and enhance overall mood.

Setting Realistic Goals:

Encourage seniors to set realistic and achievable goals for their chair yoga practice. These goals can be related to physical improvements, emotional well-being, or overall health.

4 Celebrating Achievements:

Acknowledge and celebrate small achievements. Recognizing progress, no matter how minor, motivates seniors to maintain a consistent practice by highlighting the positive impacts of their efforts.

5 Group Support and Social Engagement:

Foster a sense of community within the chair yoga group. Group support provides motivation, encouragement, and a shared commitment to regular practice.

6 Establishing a Routine:

Help seniors incorporate chair yoga into their daily or weekly routine. Establishing a regular practice time creates a sense of structure and makes it easier for participants to commit to the practice.

7 Flexibility in Scheduling:

Recognize the need for flexibility in scheduling. Seniors may have varying energy levels or external commitments, so offering flexibility in practice times accommodates individual preferences.

8 Setting Reminders:

Suggest the use of reminders, whether through alarms, calendars, or other tools. Reminders prompt seniors to prioritize their chair yoga practice and make it a consistent part of their day.

9 Tailoring Sessions to Abilities:

Customize chair yoga sessions based on individual abilities and needs. Offering personalized modifications ensures that participants can comfortably engage in the practice, fostering a sense of enjoyment and accomplishment.

Variety in Practices:

Introduce a variety of chair yoga practices to prevent monotony. Incorporate sessions focusing on balance, flexibility, strength, and relaxation to cater to different aspects of well-being.

Encouraging Self-Reflection:

Foster self-reflection within the practice. Encourage seniors to listen to their bodies, understand their limits, and adapt the practice accordingly. This self-awareness contributes to a sustainable and consistent practice

Clear Communication:

Maintain clear communication with participants. Provide guidance on the benefits of a consistent practice and offer insights into how chair yoga can positively impact their overall health.

Accessible Resources:

Provide accessible resources, such as instructional materials, videos, or online sessions, to support seniors in their home practice. Accessible resources enhance their ability to maintain consistency outside of group sessions.

Regular Check-Ins:

Conduct regular check-ins with participants to understand their experiences, address any concerns, and offer additional guidance. This personal connection strengthens the sense of community and commitment to consistent practice.

Tracking Progress:

Maintaining a Journal:

Suggest maintaining a journal to track progress. Seniors can document how they feel physically and emotionally after each session, providing a tangible record of their journey

Periodic Assessments:

Conduct periodic assessments or reviews to help seniors recognize improvements and set new goals. This reflective practice reinforces the positive impact of consistent chair yoga.

Chair yoga can be seamlessly integrated into the daily routines of seniors, offering a convenient and accessible way to promote physical and mental well-being. This subchapter explores practical strategies and considerations for incorporating chair yoga into the daily lives of seniors, emphasizing the transformative impact on their overall health.

1 Morning Chair Yoga Routine:

Gentle Wake-Up Stretches:

Begin the day with gentle chair yoga stretches. Seated neck stretches, shoulder rotations, and ankle circles help awaken the body and improve circulation.

2 Sun Salutations from the Chair:

Introduce modified sun salutations from the chair to promote flexibility and energize the body. This sequence can include seated forward bends and gentle twists.

3 Breathing Exercises for Focus:

Incorporate breath-focused exercises to enhance focus and mental clarity. Techniques like diaphragmatic breathing or alternate nostril breathing can be done comfortably in a seated position

4 Midday Relaxation Break:

Take a midday break to practice chair yoga for stress relief. Seated meditation or gentle stretches can help alleviate tension and re-energize for the rest of the day.

5 Ergonomic Seated Posture Practices:

Integrate ergonomic seated posture practices into daily activities. Seniors can practice maintaining a tall spine and engaging their core while sitting at a desk, watching TV, or reading.

6 Chair Yoga Desk Stretches:

Offer chair yoga desk stretches for seniors with sedentary jobs. Simple seated stretches and movements can be done at a desk to release tension and prevent stiffness.

7 Mindful Walking Breaks:

Encourage short mindful walking breaks. Seniors can practice walking mindfully, paying attention to each step and fostering a connection between movement and breath.

8 Evening Relaxation Ritual:

Seated Relaxation Poses:

Wind down the day with seated relaxation poses. Gentle seated forward bends and twists can help release tension and prepare the body for a restful evening.

9 Guided Meditation from the Chair:

Include guided meditation from the chair in the evening routine. This practice promotes relaxation, reduces stress, and prepares seniors for a peaceful night's sleep.

10 Breathing Techniques for Sleep:

Teach calming breathing techniques for better sleep. Slow, deep breaths or progressive relaxation can be done while seated in the evening to induce a state of calmness.

11 Daily Life Integration Strategies:

Chair Yoga While Watching TV:

Suggest incorporating chair yoga during TV time. Seniors can perform gentle stretches or seated poses while enjoying their favorite shows, making it a seamless part of their leisure activities.

12 Mindful Eating Practices:

Seniors can practice seated mindfulness while enjoying meals, focusing on the sensory experience of eating and promoting a sense of gratitude.

13 Chair Yoga as Social Activity:

Promote chair yoga as a social activity. Encourage seniors to engage in chair yoga with friends or family, creating a supportive community and making it an enjoyable shared experience

14 Individualized Short Sessions:

Emphasize the effectiveness of short, individualized chair yoga sessions. Seniors can tailor their practice based on their daily energy levels, time constraints, and specific needs.

15 Adapting Poses for Daily Ailments:

Teach seniors to adapt chair yoga poses based on daily ailments or discomfort. Offering modifications empowers them to address specific concerns and make the practice more personalized.

16 Daily Intentions and Reflections:

Encourage setting daily intentions before chair yoga sessions. Seniors can reflect on their intentions during and after practice, fostering a mindful approach and enhancing the overall impact.

CONCLUSION

Chair yoga can be seamlessly integrated into the daily routines of seniors, offering a convenient and accessible way to promote physical and mental well-being. This subchapter explores practical strategies and considerations for incorporating chair yoga into the daily lives of seniors, emphasizing the transformative impact on their overall health.

Gentle Wake-Up Stretches:

Begin the day with gentle chair yoga stretches. Seated neck stretches, shoulder rotations, and ankle circles help awaken the body and improve circulation.

Sun Salutations from the Chair:

Introduce modified sun salutations from the chair to promote flexibility and energize the body. This sequence can include seated forward bends and gentle twists.

Breathing Exercises for Focus:

Incorporate breath-focused exercises to enhance focus and mental clarity. Techniques like diaphragmatic breathing or alternate nostril breathing can be done comfortably in a seated position.

Chair Yoga for Stress Relief:

Take a midday break to practice chair yoga for stress relief. Seated meditation or gentle stretches can help alleviate tension and re-energize for the rest of the day.

Ergonomic Seated Posture Practices:

Integrate ergonomic seated posture practices into daily activities. Seniors can practice maintaining a tall spine and engaging their core while sitting at a desk, watching TV, or reading.

Chair Yoga Desk Stretches:

Offer chair yoga desk stretches for seniors with sedentary jobs. Simple seated stretches and movements can be done at a desk to release tension and prevent stiffness.

Joint Mobility Exercises:

Include joint mobility exercises in the afternoon routine. Seated joint rotations and gentle movements improve flexibility and maintain joint health.

Chair Warrior Poses:

Incorporate chair warrior poses to enhance strength and stability. These seated variations provide a beneficial workout for the lower body.

Mindful Walking Breaks:

Encourage short mindful walking breaks. Seniors can practice walking mindfully, paying attention to each step and fostering a connection between movement and breath.

Seated Relaxation Poses:

Wind down the day with seated relaxation poses. Gentle seated forward bends and twists can help release tension and prepare the body for a restful evening.

Guided Meditation from the Chair:

Include guided meditation from the chair in the evening routine. This practice promotes relaxation, reduces stress, and prepares seniors for a peaceful night's sleep.

Breathing Techniques for Sleep:

Teach calming breathing techniques for better sleep. Slow, deep breaths or progressive relaxation can be done while seated in the evening to induce a state of calmness.

Chair Yoga While Watching TV:

Suggest incorporating chair yoga during TV time. Seniors can perform gentle stretches or seated poses while enjoying their favorite shows, making it a seamless part of their leisure activities.

Mindful Eating Practices:

Introduce mindful eating practices. Seniors can practice seated mindfulness while enjoying meals, focusing on the sensory experience of eating and promoting a sense of gratitude.

Chair Yoga as Social Activity:

Promote chair yoga as a social activity. Encourage seniors to engage in chair yoga with friends or family, creating a supportive community and making it an enjoyable shared experience.

Individualized Short Sessions:

Emphasize the effectiveness of short, individualized chair yoga sessions. Seniors can tailor their practice based on their daily energy levels, time constraints, and specific needs.

Adapting Poses for Daily Ailments:

Teach seniors to adapt chair yoga poses based on daily ailments or discomfort. Offering modifications empowers them to address specific concerns and make the practice more personalized.

Daily Intentions and Reflections:

Encourage setting daily intentions before chair yoga sessions. Seniors can reflect on their intentions during and after practice, fostering a mindful approach and enhancing the overall impact.

Maintaining a Chair Yoga Journal:

Recommend maintaining a chair yoga journal. Seniors can track their daily practice, note any improvements, and reflect on the holistic benefits experienced over time.

Celebrating Milestones:

Celebrate milestones and consistent efforts. Acknowledge achievements, whether they be physical improvements, increased mindfulness, or a deeper sense of relaxation, reinforcing the positive impact of daily chair yoga.